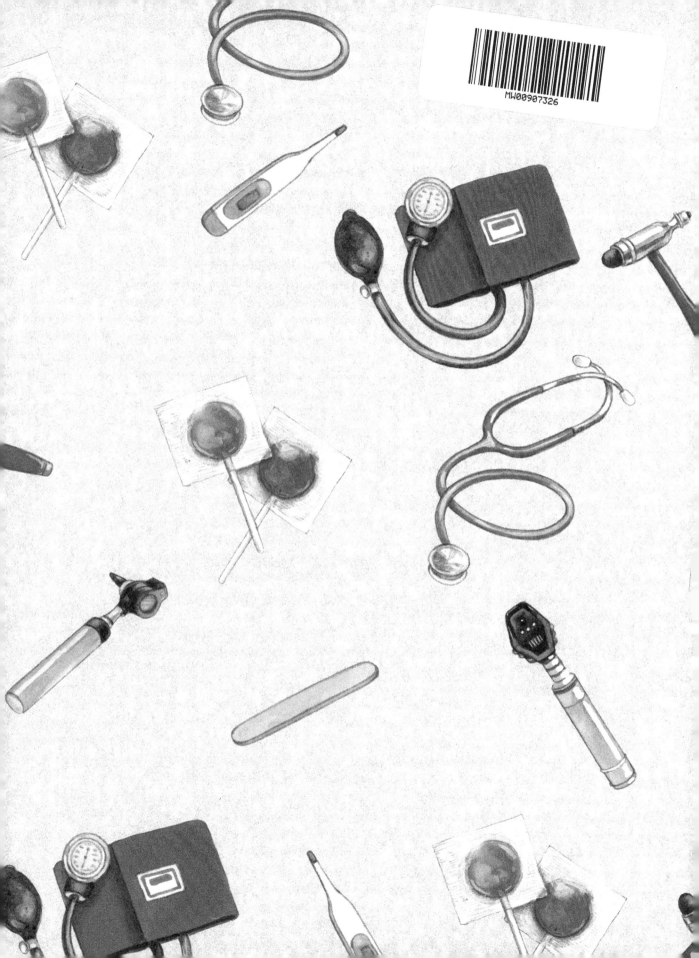

Special thanks...

To my team: Esther Hershenhorn, my forever graphic designer Aaron Morishita
and as always, to my wonderful family for their continual support.

This book is dedicated to all the parents and the children who have been
part of my life in my years as a pediatrician. It's been an honor, a privilege
and a joy to participate in your child's health care. – C.dF.

For Gage Sanders, Braveheart, truly one of the bravest kids I've ever known – T.L.

www.jakeskindergartencheckup.com

Dr. Dee's Publishing
4680 Tarantella Lane, San Diego, CA 92130
Copyright © 2016 Chrystal de Freitas with Illustrations by Tammie Lyon

A portion of the proceeds will be donated to non-profit programs for children's literacy.

Library of Congress Cataloging-in-Publication Data

De Freitas, Chrystal.
   Jake's kindergarten checkup / written by Dr. Chrystal de Freitas ; illustrated by Tammie Lyon. -- First edition.
     pages : color illustrations ; cm. -- (A sister, me and Dr. Dee book)
   Summary: "Jake welcomes his kindergarten checkup with Dr. Dee but fears the necessary inevitable shots. His tag-along sister Chloe increases his fear at each step of the exam until her surprising empathy helps Jake muster the courage to complete the checkup. The two head home, Jake kindergarten-bound, both dually-rewarded. Included: easy-to-understand explanations of a checkup's elements and the accompanying medical tools and Tips for Parents: Preparing for Your Child's Well Child Checkup and Vaccines."--Provided by publisher.
   ISBN: 978-0-9844529-4-1

   1. Vaccination--Juvenile fiction. 2. Medical care--Juvenile fiction. 3. Brothers and sisters--Juvenile fiction. 4. Physicians--Juvenile fiction. 5. Kindergarten--Juvenile fiction. 6. Medical care--Fiction. 7. Brothers and sisters--Fiction. 8. Physicians--Fiction. 9. Kindergarten--Fiction. 10. Picture books. I. Lyon, Tammie. II. Title.
PZ7.1.D44 Ja 2016
[E]
                 Library of Congress Control Number: 2015913892

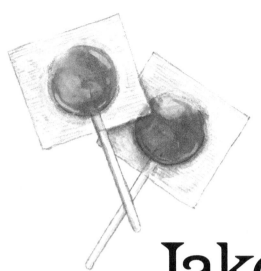

Jake's Kindergarten Checkup

MY SISTER, ME & DR. DEE BOOK 1

Written by Dr. Chrystal de Freitas
Illustrated by Tammie Lyon

Dr. Dee's Publishing
San Diego, CA

To Anika & Sam
Keeping children healthy
Dr. d
2018

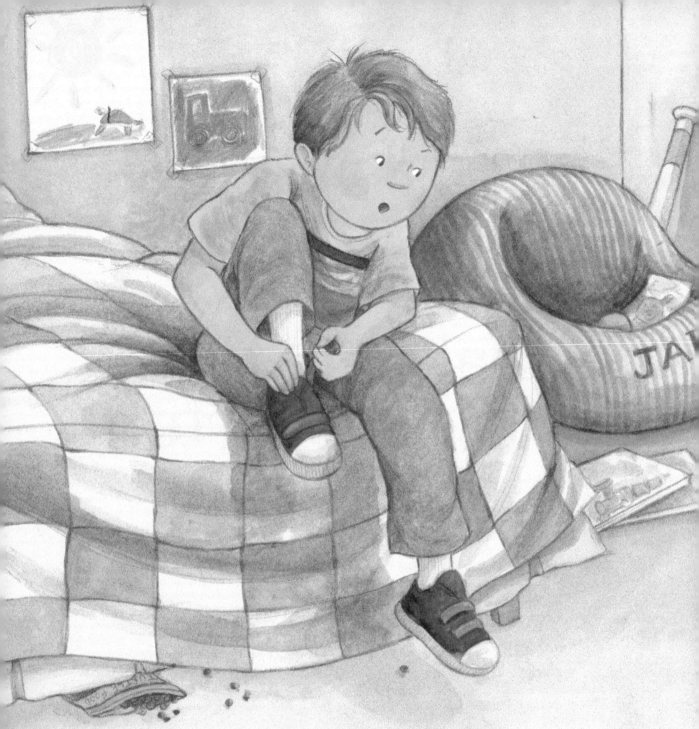

Jake was smiles all summer long. He was—*almost*—a kindergartner. He was excited to learn new things and make new friends.

But one thing worried him—a lot! Before school began he'd need his kindergarten checkup with Dr. Dee and a checkup *usually* meant shots.

"I want to come too!" his little sister Chloe begged when checkup day finally arrived. She packed up her doctor's kit and was ready to go. "Dr. Dee always gives me a princess sticker and a lollipop."

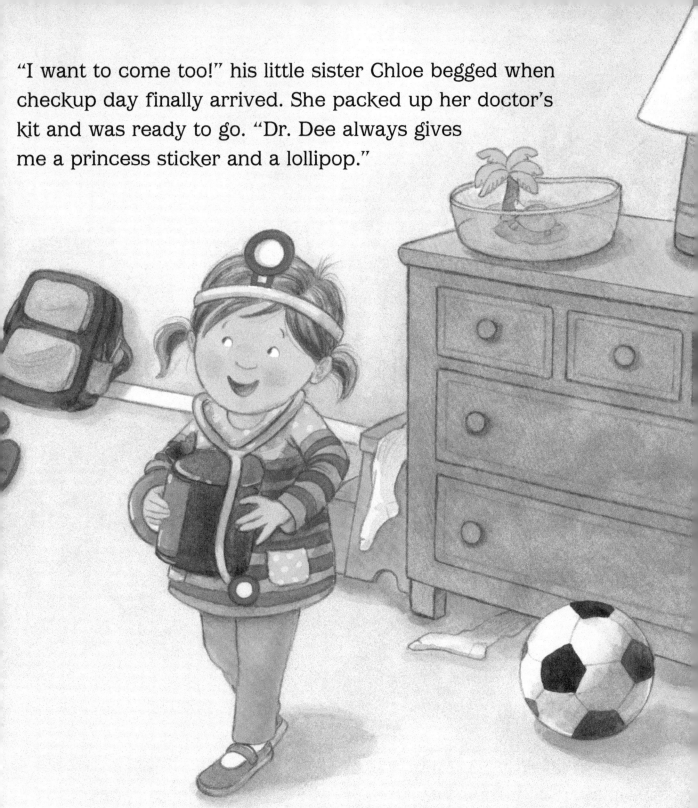

"You need to get a shot first, Chloe, to get a sticker and a lollipop," Jake replied, frowning. He couldn't shake his shot worries.

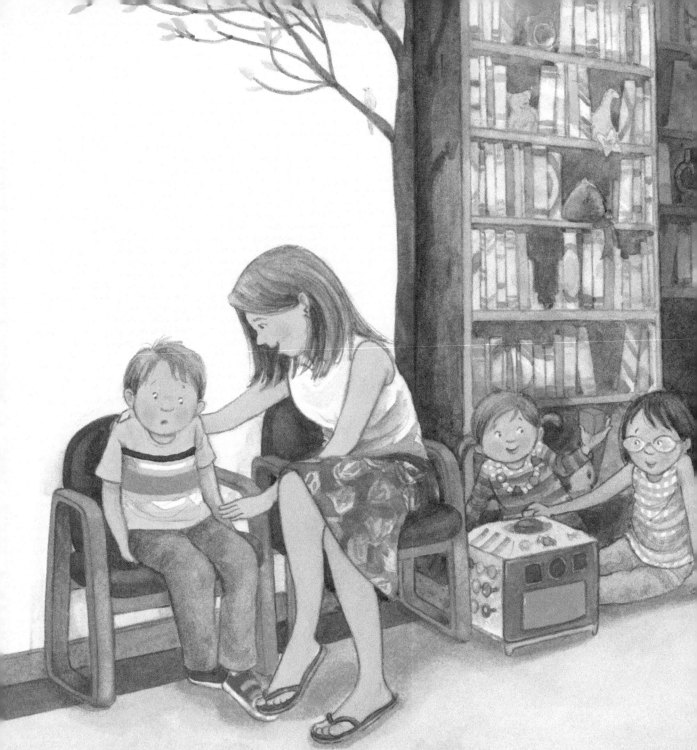

At the doctor's office, Jake waited nervously while Chloe
played with the other kids. "I'm not getting a shot today," she
announced. "Only my brother is. He's going to kindergarten."

Jake did his best to look brave, but remembered that he
cried at his last checkup visit.

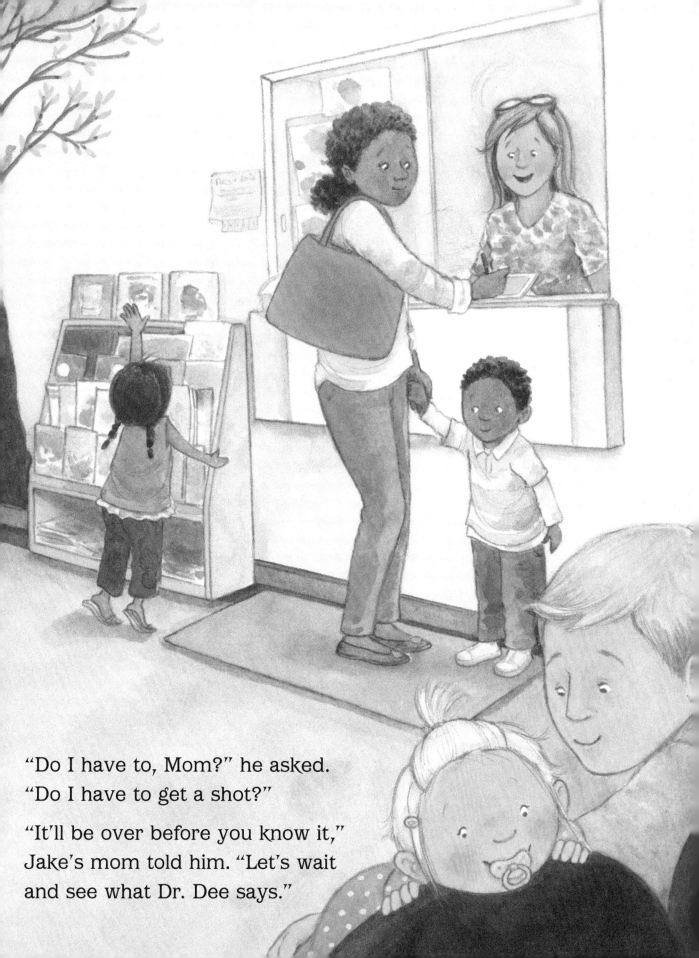

"Do I have to, Mom?" he asked.
"Do I have to get a shot?"

"It'll be over before you know it,"
Jake's mom told him. "Let's wait
and see what Dr. Dee says."

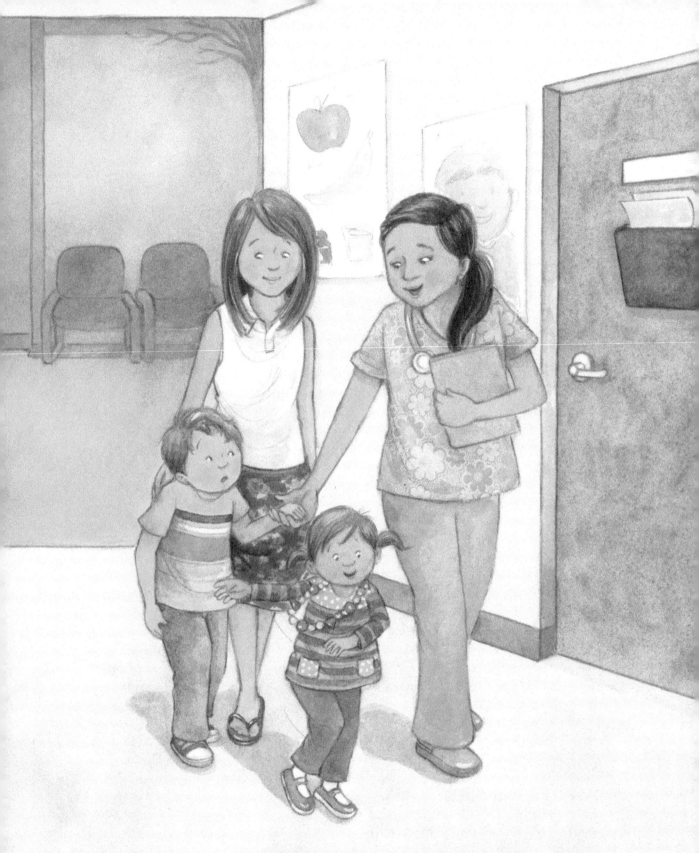

There was no turning back once Nurse Lilly called Jake's name. "Time to have some fun, kids!" she told them.

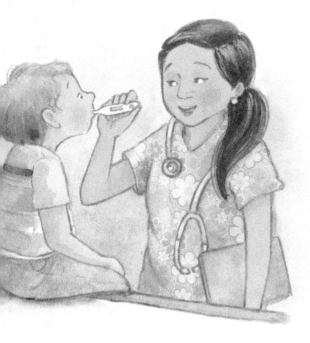

As always, Nurse Lilly took Jake's temperature.

"No fever. Perfect!" she said.

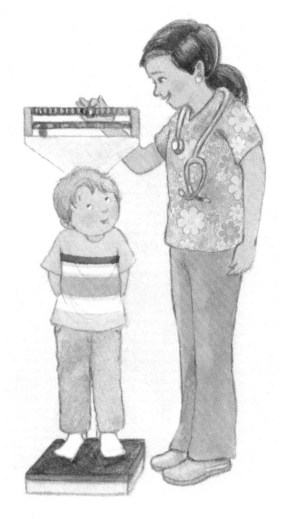

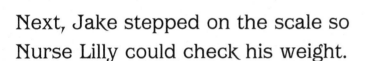

Next, Jake stepped on the scale so Nurse Lilly could check his weight.

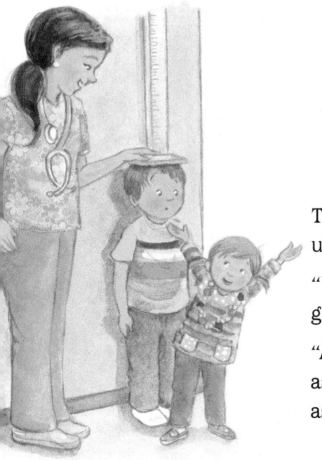

Then she measured his height using the scale's height bar.

"Wow, Jake! You sure have grown!" Nurse Lilly told him.

"And what about me?" Chloe asked. "My turn. Someday I'll be as big and tall as Jake, right?!"

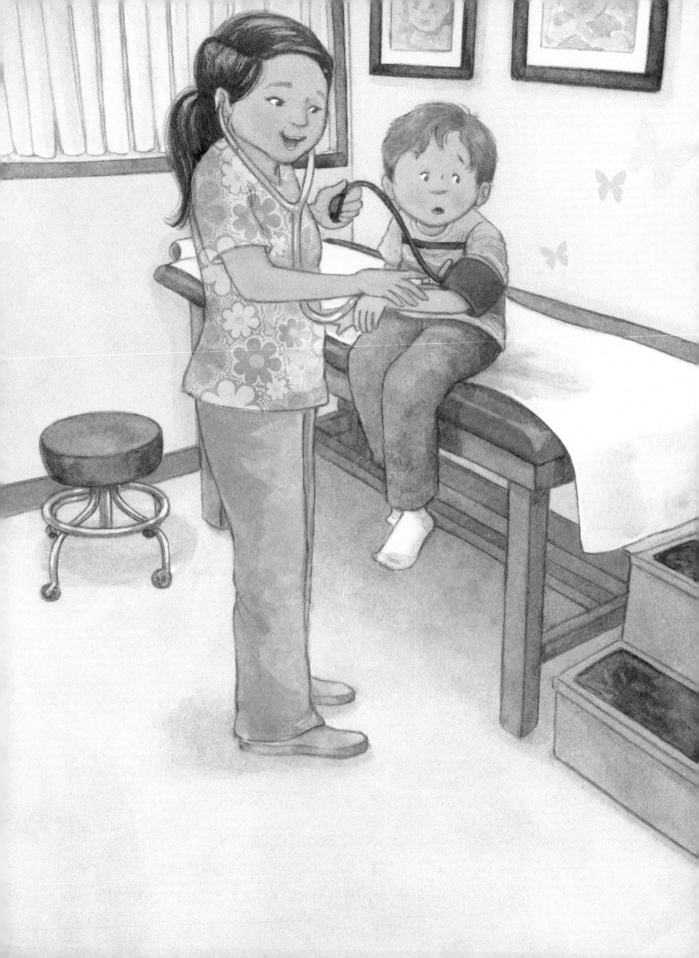

Jake climbed onto the papered examination table so Nurse Lilly could measure his blood pressure with her special cuff.

"This cuff is like a bracelet that squeezes your arm to measure how strong your heart is," she explained.

Chloe was demanding *her* turn when a baby's cry stopped her.

"Is that baby getting a shot?" Jake asked.

"Don't worry, Jake. You're not a baby," Chloe said. "You're starting kindergarten next week!"

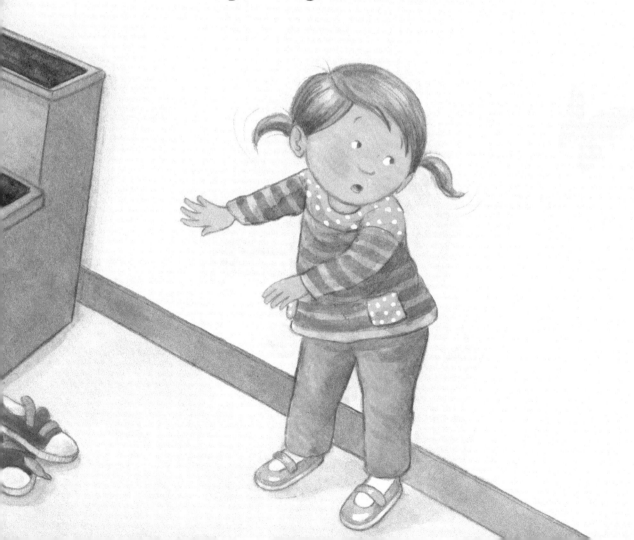

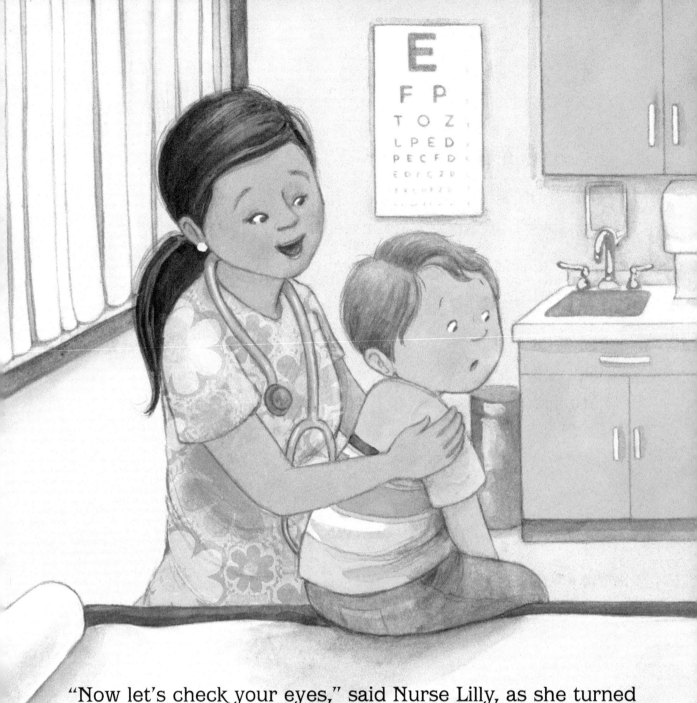

"Now let's check your eyes," said Nurse Lilly, as she turned Jake to face the eye chart so he could read the letters.

But Chloe beat him to it. "E-F-P-T-O-Z!" she shouted as she covered one eye.

"Chloe! This is my appointment. Remember?!" Jake told her, reading the letters from top to bottom.

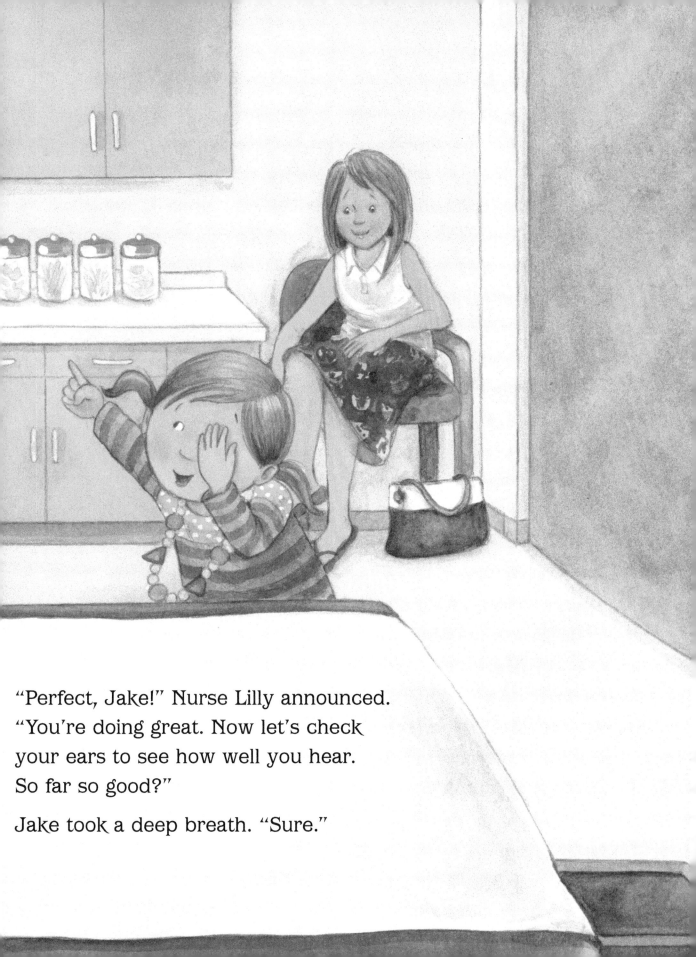

"Perfect, Jake!" Nurse Lilly announced.
"You're doing great. Now let's check
your ears to see how well you hear.
So far so good?"

Jake took a deep breath. "Sure."

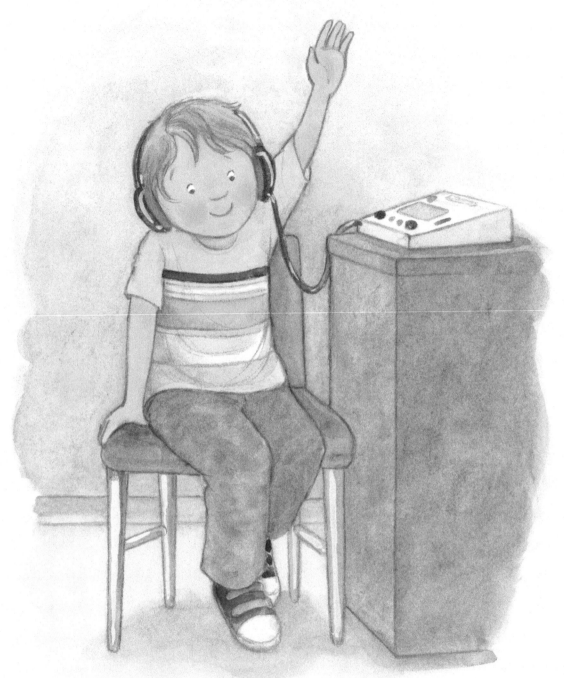

Chloe laughed when Nurse Lilly pronounced the sound machine's strange name—*audiometer*.

"Shhhh!" Jake told her, putting on his earphones. "I need to listen." He raised his right arm each time he heard the machine's *peep*.

"Perfect!" Nurse Lilly said.

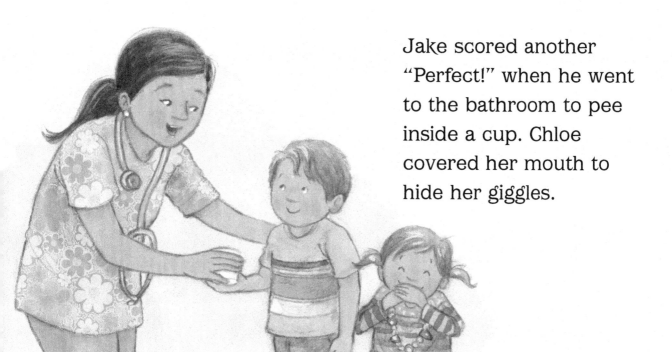

Jake scored another "Perfect!" when he went to the bathroom to pee inside a cup. Chloe covered her mouth to hide her giggles.

"The correct word for pee is *urine,*" Nurse Lilly explained. "Believe it or not, checking your urine tells us just how well the inside of your body is working."

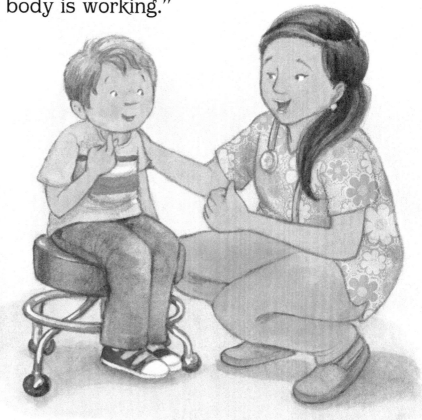

"Are we done now?" Jake asked Nurse Lilly, crossing his fingers.

"My part is, so good luck in kindergarten! Now it's time to see Dr. Dee."

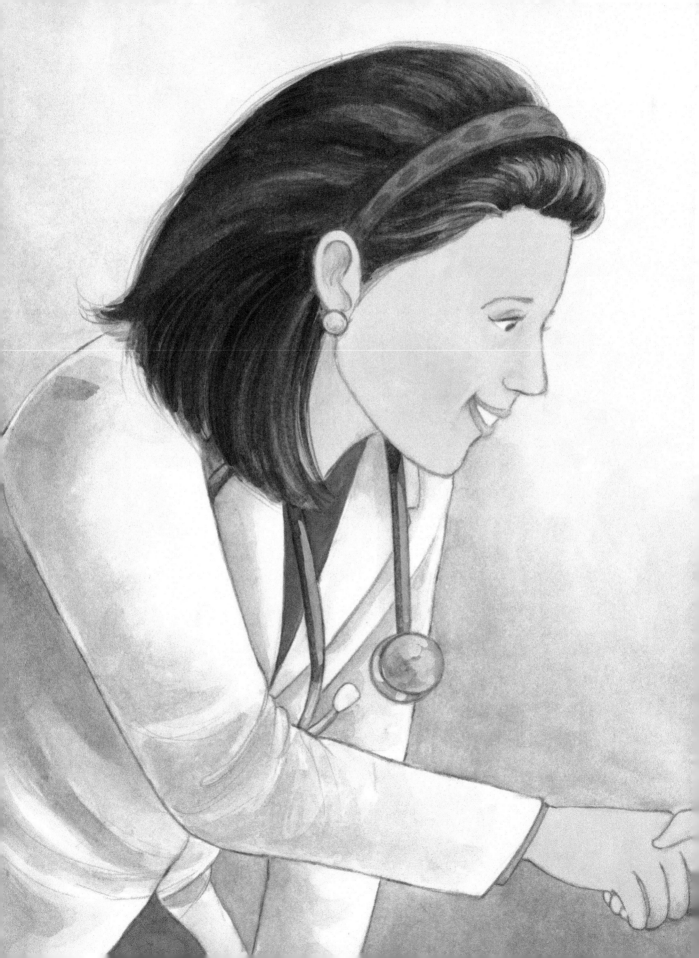

"Hi, I hear someone's ready for kindergarten," Dr. Dee announced, shaking Jake's hand and winking at Chloe. "My, how time flies!"

"And it's flying for me, too?" Chloe asked.

"For sure," said Dr. Dee.

"I got lots of 'Perfects!' from Nurse Lilly... so I don't need any shots. Right?" asked Jake.

"Well, Jake, let's first take a look and a listen and check out how you're doing."

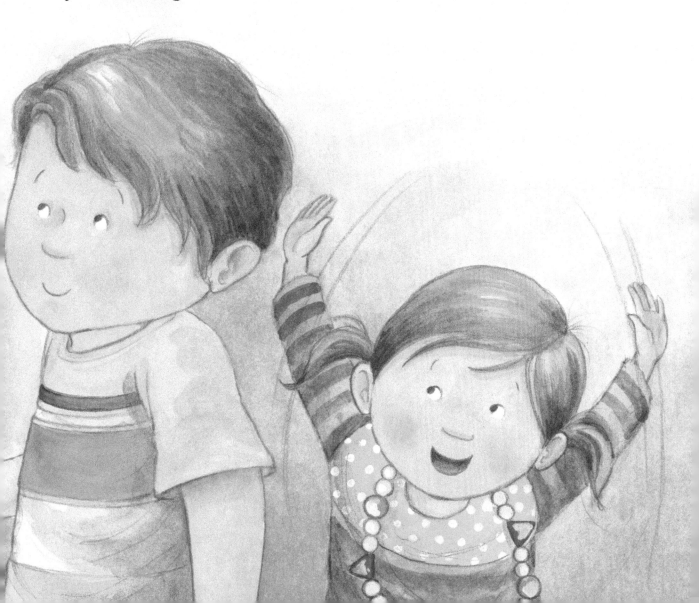

Dr. Dee examined Jake from head to toe. She used all sorts of funny-looking instruments with hard-to-pronounce names. Chloe wanted to see everything.

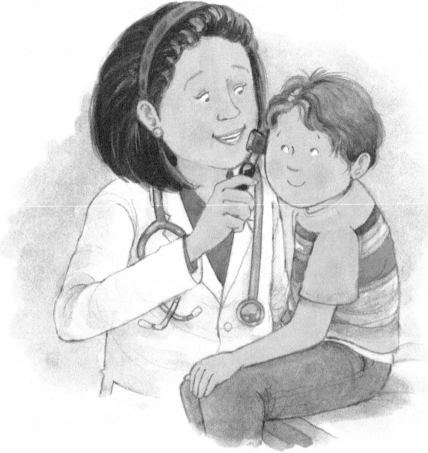

First, Dr. Dee checked Jake's ears with her *otoscope*.

Next, she checked Jake's eyes with her *ophthalmoscope*.

"When is it my turn?" Chloe asked again and again. "Can I see?"

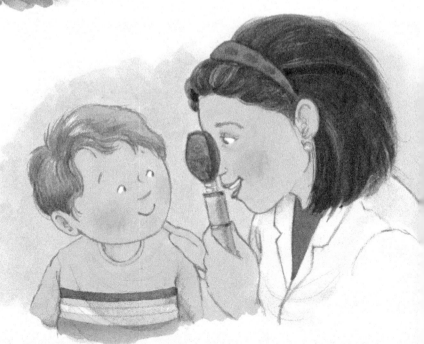

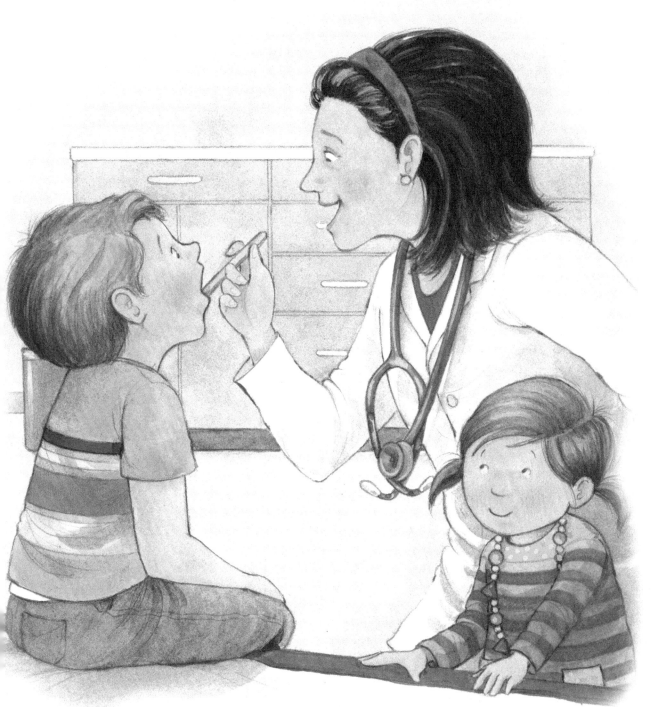

"Say, 'Ahhhhh'," Dr. Dee told Jake. She used her *tongue depressor* to hold Jake's tongue still so she could see all the way to the back of his mouth.

Jake took a big breath. "I'm sure glad I'm not getting any shots today, Dr. Dee."

"Me too," Chloe added.

"Have you ever listened to your own heart beat, Jake?" Dr. Dee asked. She used her *stethoscope* to listen to Jake's heart. Then she placed its earpieces in Jake's ears so he could listen too.

"What's it saying?" Chloe asked. "Can I listen?"

"Lub-dub, lub-dub, lub-dub," Jake told her.
"Like a drum beat!"

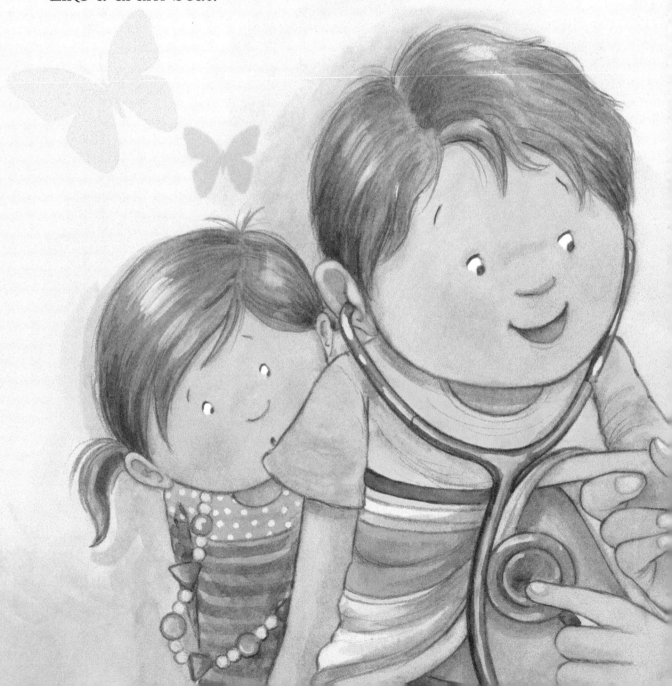

"So, now it's time for Jake's shots?" Chloe asked.

Jake was so distracted listening to his heart beat that he didn't even hear her.

But there was still more for Dr. Dee to check.

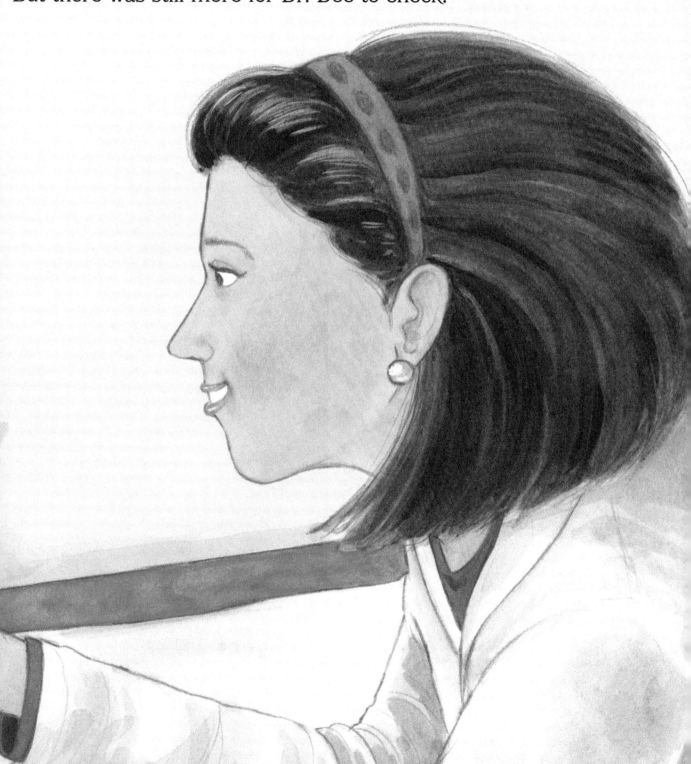

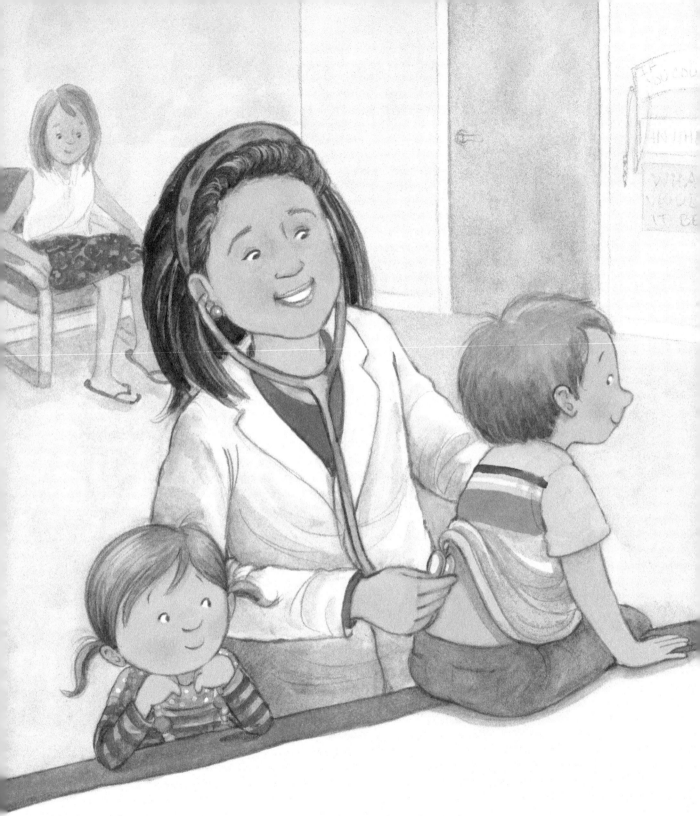

Now it was time for Dr. Dee to check Jake's lungs.

"Take a deep breath, Jake," she repeated as she moved the stethoscope across his back.

Next Jake laid down so Dr. Dee could use her stethoscope to listen to his tummy. She even poked his belly with her fingers.

"Did you have waffles for breakfast?" Dr. Dee teased.

Jake and Chloe were full of giggles!

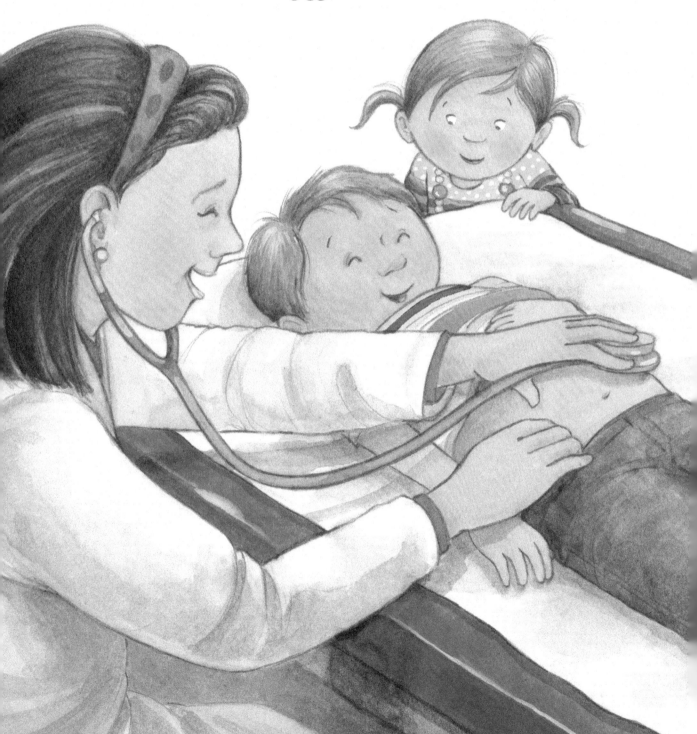

"Finally!" Jake said, sitting up. "This is my favorite part."

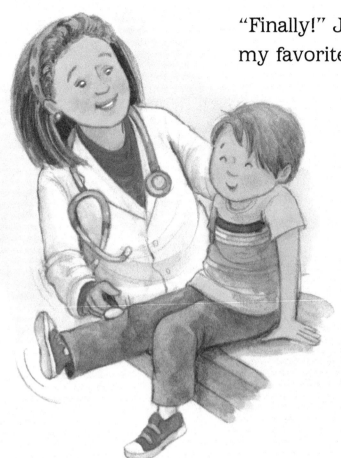

Dr. Dee used her *reflex hammer* to tap below his right knee.

Pop! Out swung Jake's right foot.

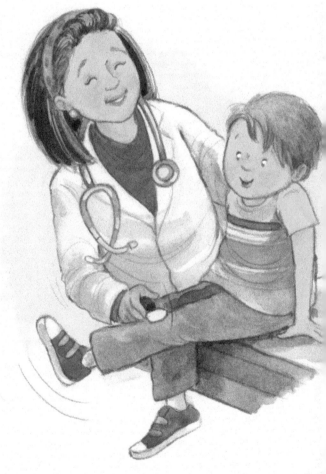

His left foot did the same when she tapped below his left knee.

"You are the picture of health, Jake!" Dr. Dee said. "Thanks, Mom, for helping Jake stay healthy."

"So if everything is perfect I don't need a shot, right?"
Jake asked. He smiled nervously.

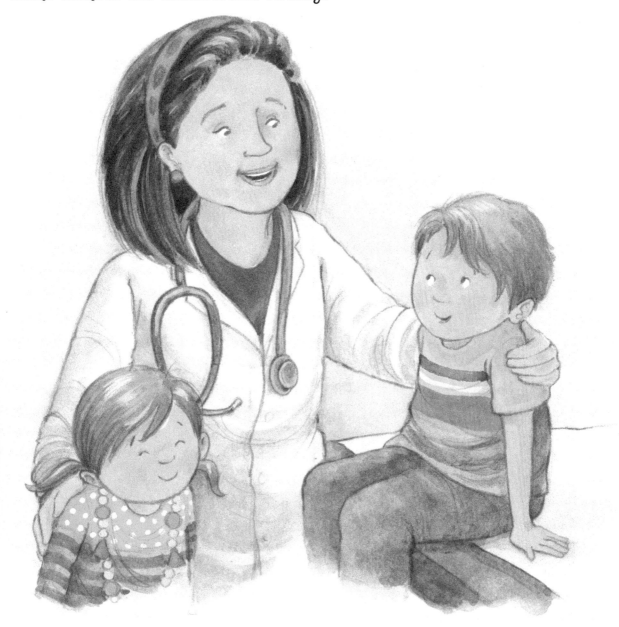

"Just about all my patients hate getting shots," said Dr. Dee,
"but a shot helps your body fight germs so you can stay
healthy. A shot is really just a small needle that gives your
body a special medicine to help protect it from diseases
like measles and whooping cough. That way you can stay
strong and healthy."

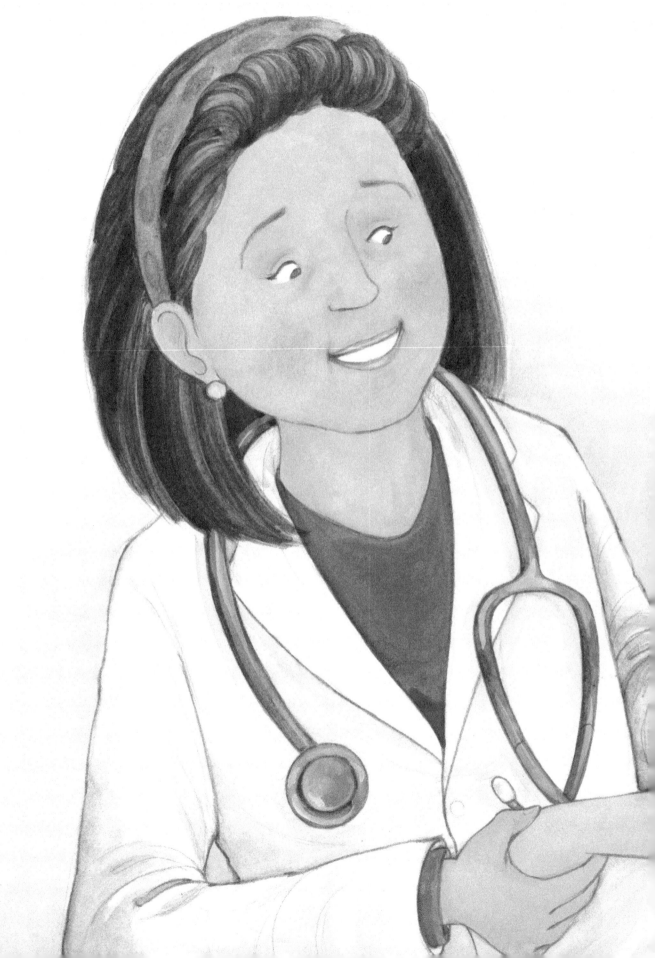

Jake closed his right eye tight, scrunched his lips and braced himself for what was coming next. But to everyone's surprise, Chloe began to cry. She bawled!!

"My brother and I don't like shots!" she shouted.
"We want to go home!"

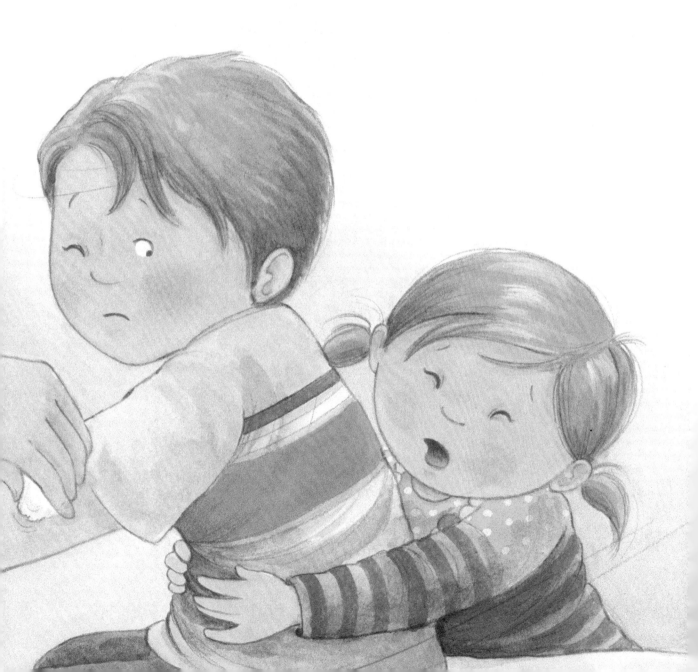

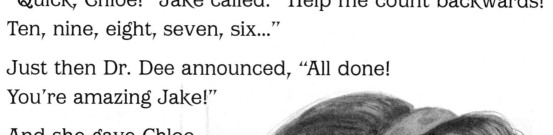

"Quick, Chloe!" Jake called. "Help me count backwards! Ten, nine, eight, seven, six..."

Just then Dr. Dee announced, "All done! You're amazing Jake!"

And she gave Chloe a special wink.

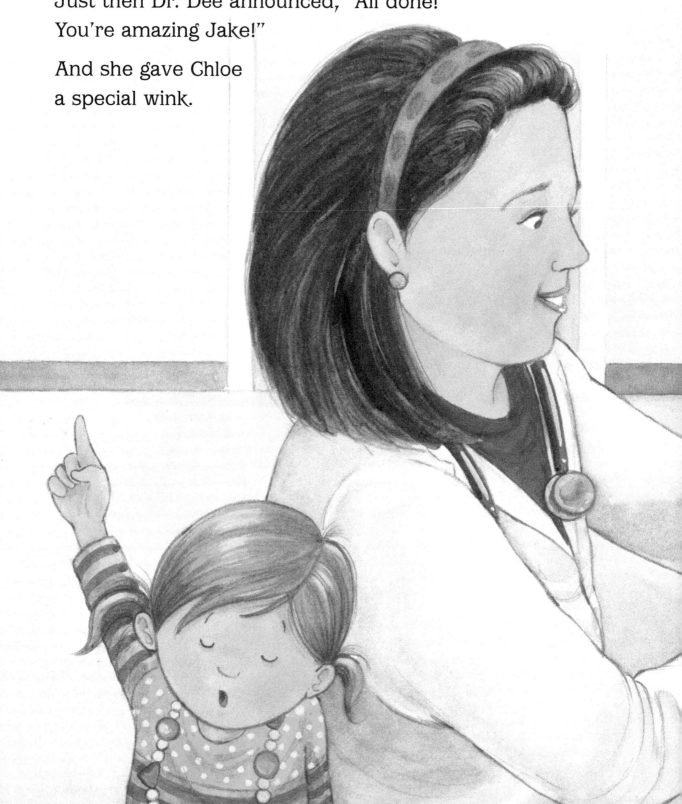

"Did it hurt, did it hurt?" Chloe wanted to know.

"Hardly at all thanks to you," Jake answered. "I'll help you when it's your turn, Chloe."

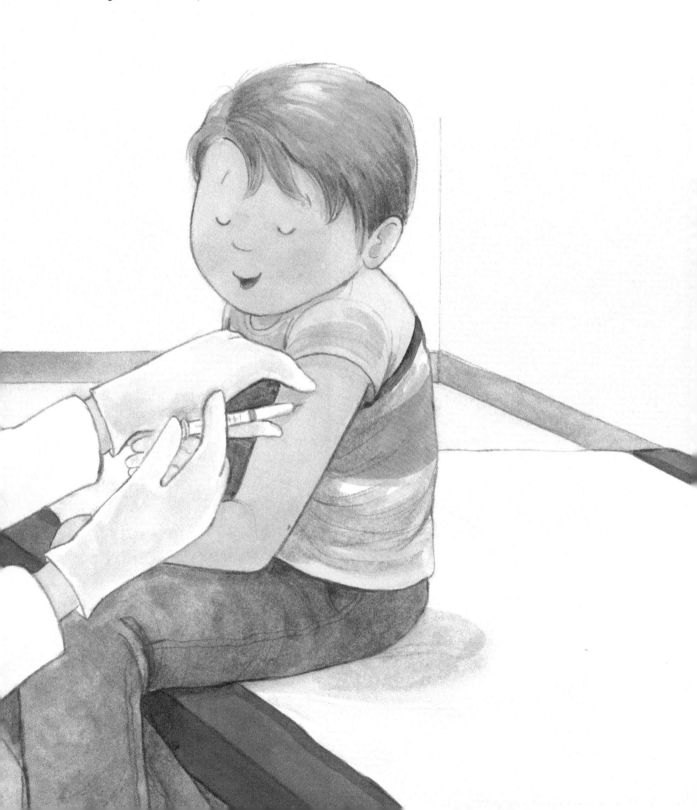

Jake asked Dr. Dee for two lollipops—cherry for him and orange for Chloe.

"Plus a princess sticker for my helper, please?" he asked.

"Of course," said Dr. Dee. "How could I say NO to such a brave and healthy kindergartner?"

Once again, Jake was all smiles.

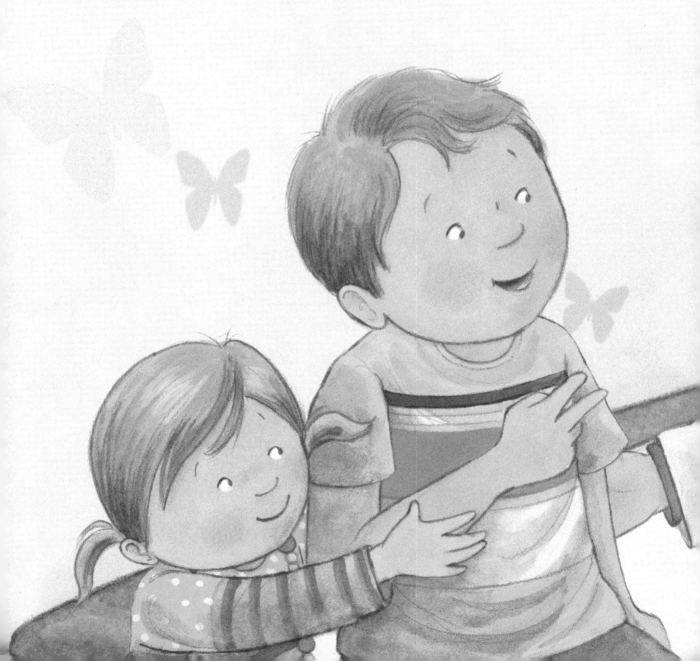

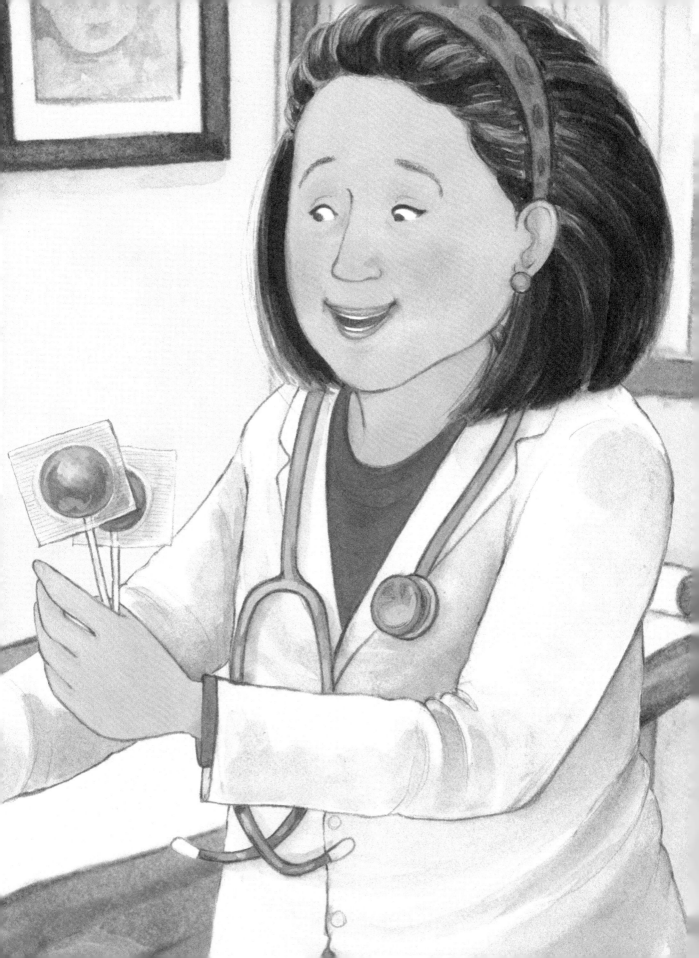

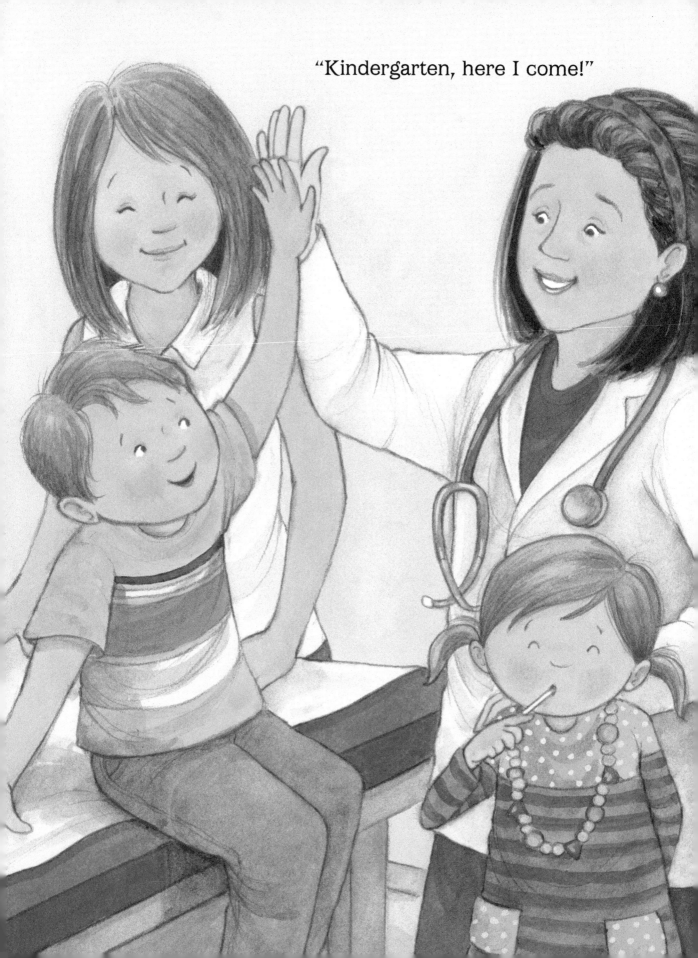

"Kindergarten, here I come!"

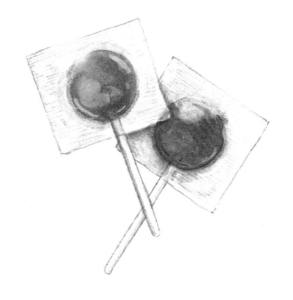

About the Author

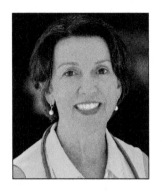

Dr. Chrystal de Freitas is an author, mother and pediatrician with a special interest in health education. While *Jake's Kindergarten Checkup* is her first picture book, she has authored several other well-received books and educational material in her field. A pediatrician for over 34 years, Dr. de Freitas is the founder of Carmel Valley Pediatrics. In addition, she is the President of Healthy Chats® which provides health education seminars to parents and their pre-teen children in the community, at the local hospitals and online. Among her honors and achievements, she has been selected by the San Diego County Medical Society and *San Diego Magazine* as one of the area's top doctors. Dr. de Freitas lives in San Diego, California, with her husband, Dr. Jeffrey Bonadio. They have three adult children.

About the Illustrator

Tammie Lyon is the award-winning author and illustrator of numerous books for children. *Let's Hear It For Almigal* was recently awarded the Mom's Choice Award Gold Medal Winner. *My Pup* and *Bugs In My Hair,* have both been included on the list of the "Top 100 Best Children's Books" by the Bank Street College of Education and The *Channing O'Banning* series was awarded the Ben Franklin award for excellence in independent publishing. She is known for her work on 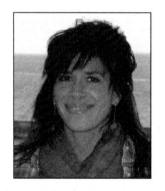 the *Eloise* series for Simon and Schuster as well as her new series, *Katie Woo,* published by Stonearch Books. Tammie's first written and illustrated title, *Olive and Snowflake,* Marshall Cavendish Publisher, has been released receiving starred reviews from both Kirkus and School Library Journal. Tammie is currently writing and illustrating an early chapter series for emergent readers which she has developed to celebrate children's diversity.

Dr. Dee's Well Child Checkup Tips for Parents

Routine Well Child Checkups are important! They help health care providers keep track of your child's growth, development and immunizations.

To make sure your child's Well Child Checkup visit goes well:

- Let your child know about the checkup beforehand. Use your best judgement as to *just* how long beforehand.

- Cast the office visit in a positive light—it's all about staying healthy!

- Help your child "play out" the visit ahead of time with a Doctor's Kit or the reading of a book, such as this one, about a checkup.

- Arrive early so you have time to fill out the necessary paper work and your child can play in the Waiting Area.

- Assure your child that shots keep the body healthy and the health care provider chooses the shots that are best.

- Reassure your child calmly that you're aware that shots hurt, but on a scale of 0 to 10, the pain will be about a "3." Counting backwards from 10 also helps.

- Plan time to celebrate the completion of the checkup!

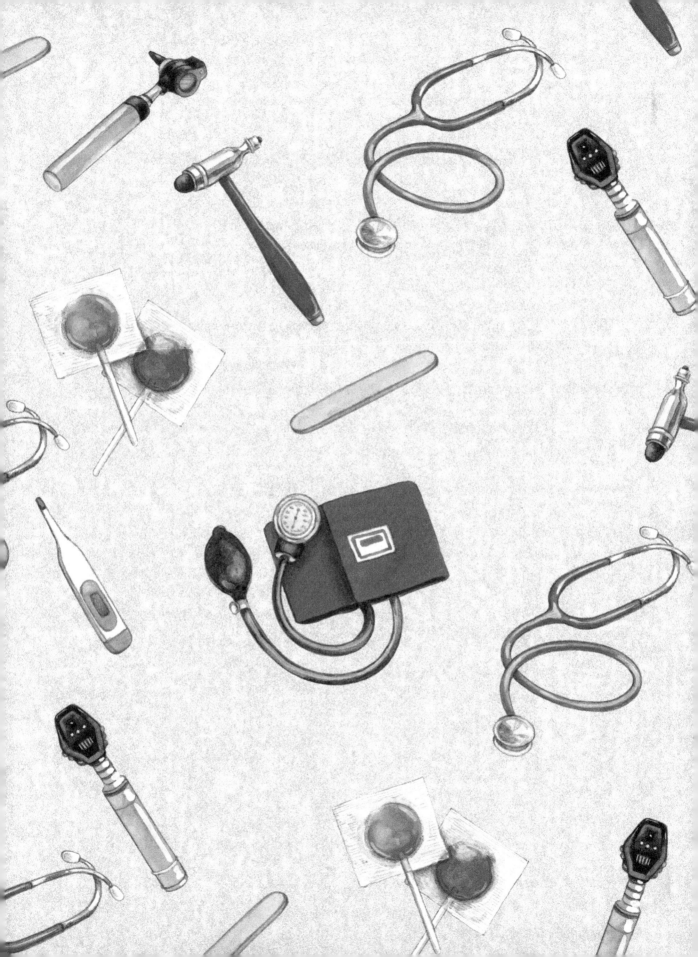

CPSIA information can be obtained
at www.ICGtesting.com
Printed in the USA
LVOW06s0449031017
550799LV00005B/35/P

Jake's Kindergarten Checkup

Jake welcomes his kindergarten checkup with Dr. Dee but fears the necessary and inevitable shots. His tag-along sister Chloe increases his fear at each step of the exam until her surprising empathy helps Jake muster the courage to complete the checkup. The two head home, Jake kindergarten-bound, both deliciously rewarded.

Includes easy-to-understand explanations of a checkup's elements and accompanying medical tools and tips that help you prepare for your child's well checkup and vaccines.

"Starting kindergarten is a huge milestone in a child's life and Dr. de Freitas' book about preparing for this school checkup is a valuable tool for parents, children and healthcare providers."

—Linda Jonides, BS, RN, CPNP

The My Sister, Me & Dr. Dee series is dedicated to helping children and parents through difficult situations. Follow us at JakesKindergartenCheckup.com.

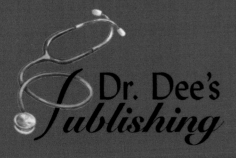
Dr. Dee's Publishing

$9.95
ISBN 978-0-9844529-4-1
50995>
9 780984 452941